30 days
KETOGENIC
cookbook

lunch edition

high fat low carb recipes for the keto diet

Recipes365

Copyright © 2017

Recipes365 Cookbooks

All rights reserved. No part of this publication may be reproduced, distributed, or transmitted in any form or by any means, including photocopying, recording, or other electronic or mechanical methods, without the prior written permission of the publisher, except in the case of brief quotations embodied in critical reviews and certain other non-commercial uses permitted by copyright law.

• BEFORE YOU BEGIN •

FREE BONUS GUIDE: TOP 10 KETO DIET MISTAKES

We've put together a free companion guide to go with this recipe book. It features the top 10 mistakes made by people on the ketogenic diet.

If you want to avoid costly mistakes and accelerate your progress you will find a link to the guide at the back of this book. If you can't wait that long, see below now!

Visit http://geni.us/ketomistakes to get your copy now!

TABLE OF CONTENTS

Introduction 1
   The Science in a Nutshell 1
   What Keto Can do for You 1
   Things to Remember 2

The Recipes 3
   Keto Flat Bread 6
   Zucchini Boats 7
   Keto Stromboli 8
   Keto Chicken Sandwich 9
   Tuna Bites with Avocado 10
   Keto Green Salad 11
   Original Keto Stuffed Hot Dogs 12
   Easy Egg Soup 13
   Original Nasi Lemak 14
   Keto Sausage and Pepper Soup 15
   Mug Cake with Jalapeño 16
   Fresh Keto Sandwich 17
   Original Squash Lasagna 18
   Chili Soup 19
   Chicken Nuggets for Keto Nuts 20
   Cauliflower Rice with Chicken 21
   Zucchini Keto Wraps 22

Cauliflower Soup with Bacon and Cheddar 23
Keto Casserole with Chicken and Bacon 24
Mexican-Style Casserole with Spinach 25
Almond Pizza 26
Chicken Salad 27
Keto Chicken Thighs 28
BBQ Chicken Soup 29
Keto Pork Stew 29
Keto Enchilada Soup 31
Grilled Cheese Sandwich 32
Keto Caprese Salad 33
Asian Salad 34
Vegetarian Curry 35

Introduction

Hello there!

Welcome to a wonderful 30 ketogenic lunches! By now you are probably well aware of the benefits of going keto but just in case you need to refresh your memory, here's a quick top-up before we dive right into the recipes.

The Science in a Nutshell

Your body normally converts carbohydrates to glucose for energy. By limiting your intake and replacing it with fats, your body enters a state of ketosis.

Here your body produces ketones, created by a breakdown of fats in the liver. Without carbohydrates as your primary source of energy your body will turn to the ketones instead.

This effectively cranks up the fat burning furnace and puts your body in the ultimate metabolic state.

What Keto Can do for You

Keto has its origins in treating healthcare conditions such as epilepsy, type 2 diabetes, cardiovascular disease, metabolic syndrome, auto-brewery syndrome and high blood pressure but now has much wider application in weight control.

This diet, then, will take you above and beyond typical results and propel you into a new realm of total body health. If you want to look and feel the best you possibly can, all without sacrificing your love of delicious food, then this is the cookbook for you.

THINGS TO REMEMBER

A healthy diet is not solution to anything in and of itself; it must be applied as part of a healthy lifestyle in order to see maximum results.

Think of the ketogenic diet as the foundation of your new body. If you want to build something truly special on top of it then design your lifestyle with that goal in mind.

Cutting out junk food goes without saying, as does ditching bad habits such as smoking and drinking. Exercise, too, will take you to heights you never thought was possible.

So, as you explore these delectable dishes and embark on the keto diet, try not to neglect other areas or responsibility.

Let this be the start of something great!

The Recipes

We wanted to make it as simple as possible for you to get in the kitchen and rustle up something special, so you will find each recipe laid out in an easy to follow format.

Each begins with a short intro to the dish, followed by the serving size and list of ingredients. Remember, this diet is designed to rekindle your love of food not extinguish it with rules and regulations, so don't be afraid to experiment.

Use the ingredients as general guidelines and follow the instructions as best you can. You may not get everything perfect first time, every time but that is what makes it yours!

Keep at it for a full 30 days of eating and you will no doubt establish a few firm favorites that you can turn into your specialty dishes over time.

Each recipe ends with a breakdown of key nutritional information including number of calories and amount of fats, carbohydrates and protein.

Again, this isn't to be obsessed over. Food is something to be enjoyed, so if you are going to keep note of your intake levels then just make it a general estimate.

Why no pics? This cookbook is full of *fun* and *flavor*, and doesn't take itself too seriously. The food is entering your mouth, not a modeling contest, and we don't like to encourage unhealthy obsession about presentation. So just cook, experiment, and enjoy.

Once you start loving what you are eating mealtimes will become something to look forward to. Take this as encouragement, go forth and cook to your heart's content!

Lunches

Keto Flat Bread

SERVES 8

For the Crust:

2 cups half-and-half grated mozzarella cheese

2 tbsp. cream cheese

¾ cup almond flour

½ tsp. sea salt

⅛ tsp. dried thyme

For the Topping:

1 cup grated Mexican cheese

½ red onion, small and sliced

4 oz. low carbohydrate sliced ham, cut

¼ medium apple, unpeeled and sliced

⅛ tsp. thyme, dried

Salt and pepper

A classic recipe that will become part of your go-to lunches. This easy recipe has apples, ham and onions – a delicious pizza style combination that you *need* to try!

1. Fill a saucepan with a little water and bring to the boil, then turn the heat to low. Place the saucepan inside a metal mixing bowl to form a double boiler, and add the mozzarella cheese, cream cheese, almond flour, thyme and salt. Stir with a spatula.
2. Cook until the cheese melts, and mix the ingredients into a dough. Pour some onto a 12-inch pizza tray covered with parchment paper. Roll the dough into a ball and place onto the center of the parchment paper. Pat into a disc shape to cover the pan.
3. Place the dough and the parchment paper on the pizza pan, poking holes throughout the dough with a fork, and bake for 6-8 minutes at 425°F. Remove.
4. Spread the toppings over the flatbread, along with the cheese, onion, apple and the ham. Cover with more cheese. Season with thyme, salt and pepper.
5. Bake again at 350°F for 5-7 minutes. Remove once the cheese begins to brown. Let cool before slicing.

NUTRITIONAL INFO PER SERVING

Calories: 257

Fat: 22g

Net Carbs: 5g

Protein: 18g

Zucchini Boats

SERVES 1

2 large zucchini

2 tbsp. butter

3 oz. shredded cheddar cheese

1 cup broccoli

6 oz. shredded rotisserie chicken

1 stalk green onion

2 tbsp. sour cream

Salt and pepper

This stuffed zucchini is an amazing option for a fast and tasty lunch packed with protein.

1. Cut the zucchini in half lengthwise, scooping out the core until you are left with a boat shape.

2. Into each zucchini pour a little melted butter, season and place into the oven at 400°F, baking for about 18 minutes.

3. In a bowl, combine the chicken, broccoli and sour cream.

4. Place the chicken mixture inside the hollowed zucchinis.

5. Top with cheddar cheese and bake for an additional 10-15 minutes.

NUTRITIONAL INFO PER SERVING

Calories: 480

Fat: 35g

Net Carbs: 5g

Protein: 28g

Keto Stromboli

Serves 4

1¼ cup shredded mozzarella cheese

4 tbsp. almond flour

3 tbsp. coconut flour

1 egg

1 tsp. Italian seasoning

4 oz. ham

4 oz. cheddar cheese

Salt and pepper

Stromboli is a traditional Italian recipe that resembles folded pizza. This keto ham and cheese version is sure to delight.

1. Melt the mozzarella cheese in the microwave for about 1 minute, stirring occasionally so as not to burn it.
2. In a separate bowl, mix almond flour, coconut flour, salt, and pepper and add the melted mozzarella cheese. Mix well. Then, after letting it cool down a bit, add the eggs and combine again.
3. Place the mixture on parchment paper, laying a second layer on top. Using your hands or rolling pin, flatten it out into a rectangle.
4. Remove the top layer of paper and with a knife cut diagonal lines toward the middle of the dough. They should be cut ⅓ of the way in on one side. Then, cut diagonal lines on the other side too.
5. On the top of the dough, alternate slices of ham and cheese. Then, fold one side over, and then the other, to cover the filling.
6. Place on a baking sheet and bake at 400°F for 15-20 minutes.

NUTRITIONAL INFO PER SERVING

Calories: 305

Fat: 22g

Net Carbs: 5g

Protein: 25g

Keto Chicken Sandwich

Serves 2

For the Bread:

3 eggs

3 oz. cream cheese

⅛ tsp. cream of tartar

Salt

Garlic powder

For the Filling:

1 tbsp. mayonnaise

1 tsp. sriracha

2 slices bacon

3 oz. chicken

2 slices pepper jack cheese

2 grape tomatoes

Make plain keto cloud bread into a sumptuous chicken sandwich. Bacon and avocado make it even more heavenly.

1. Separate the eggs in different bowls. In the egg whites add cream tartar, salt and beat until stiff peaks form.

2. In another bowl, beat the egg yolks with cream cheese. Incorporate the mixture into the egg white mixture and combine carefully.

3. Place the batter on a parchment paper and form little square shapes that look like bread slices. Sparkle garlic powder on top and bake at 300°F for 25 minutes.

4. While the bread is baking, cook the chicken and bacon in a frying pan, seasoning to taste.

5. When the bread is done, remove from oven and let cool for 10-15 minutes. Then, make the sandwich with the cooked chicken and bacon, adding the mayo, sriracha, tomatoes, cheese and mashed avocado to taste.

NUTRITIONAL INFO PER SERVING

Calories: 360

Fat: 28g

Net Carbs: 3g

Protein: 22g

Tuna Bites with Avocado

SERVES 8

10 oz. drained canned tuna

¼ cup mayo

1 avocado

¼ cup parmesan cheese

⅓ cup almond flour

½ tsp. garlic powder

¼ tsp. onion powder

½ cup coconut oil

Salt and pepper

These unique tuna bites can be served alongside a fresh salad. The avocado packs a fantastic Omega 3 fat punch!

1. In a bowl mix all the ingredients (except coconut oil). Form little balls and cover with almond flour.

2. Fry them in a pan medium heat with melted coconut oil (it has to be hot) until they seem browned on all sides.

NUTRITIONAL INFO PER SERVING

Calories: 137

Fat: 12g

Net Carbs: 10g

Protein: 6g

Keto Green Salad

SERVES 1

2 oz. mixed greens

3 tbsp. roasted pine nuts

2 tbsp. raspberry vinaigrette

2 tbsp. parmesan, shaved

2 slices bacon

Salt and pepper

Who said green salad has to be dull? These ingredients and the heavenly dressing will make your day.

1. Cook the bacon in a pan until crunchy and well browned. Break up into pieces, and add to the rest of the ingredients in a bowl.

2. Dress the salad with the raspberry vinaigrette.

NUTRITIONAL INFO PER SERVING

Calories: 480

Fat: 37g

Net Carbs: 4g

Protein: 17g

Original Keto Stuffed Hot Dogs

SERVES 6

6 hot dogs

12 slices bacon

2 oz. cheddar

½ tsp. cheese garlic powder

½ tsp. onion powder

Salt and pepper

Have just 10 minutes for lunch? No worries, this original recipe is here to help you out!

1. Make a little slit in each hot dog, and stuff them with slices of cheese. Wrap each hot dog with 2 slices of overlapping bacon, and secure with toothpicks.

2. On top of a wire rack (with a cookie sheet below), place the hotdogs. Season them and bake at 400°F for 20-25 minutes approx.

NUTRITIONAL INFO PER SERVING

Calories: 385

Fat: 34g

Net Carbs: 0.5g

Protein: 17g

Easy Egg Soup

SERVES 1

1½ cups chicken broth

½ cube of chicken bouillon

1 tbsp. bacon fat

2 eggs

1 tsp. chili garlic paste

5 minutes and 5 ingredients can make magic stuff—like this yummy egg soup.

1. In a pan on the stove on a medium-high heat, add the chicken broth, bouillon cube and bacon fat. Bring into boil and incorporate chili garlic paste and mix.

2. Whisk the eggs and add them to the chicken while stirring, then let sit for a few minutes.

NUTRITIONAL INFO PER SERVING

Calories: 280

Fat: 25g

Net Carbs: 2.7g

Protein: 13g

Original Nasi Lemak

SERVES 2

For the Chicken & Egg:

2 chicken thighs, boneless

½ tsp. curry powder

¼ tsp. turmeric powder

½ tsp. lime juice

½ tbsp. coconut oil

1 egg

A pinch of salt

For the Nasi Lemak:

3 tbsp. coconut milk

3 slices ginger

½ small shallot

1 cup riced cauliflower

4 slices cucumber

Salt

A food with Indonesian origin, this dish will crown your lunch. It may seem complicated, but it's not too hard; and it will impress, so invite a friend to join you!

1. Rice the cauliflower and strain the water.

2. Prepare the curry powder, turmeric powder, lemon juice and salt, and marinate the chicken thighs for an hour or two in the fridge. Remove and fry.

3. Boil the coconut milk, ginger and shallot in a saucepan. When it bubbles, incorporate the cauliflower rice and mix.

4. Serve with the marinated fried chicken and fried egg.

NUTRITIONAL INFO PER SERVING

Calories: 502

Fat: 40g

Net Carbs: 7g

Protein: 28g

Keto Sausage and Pepper Soup

SERVES 6

30 oz. pork sausage

1 tbsp. olive oil

10 oz. raw spinach

1 medium green bell pepper

1 can tomatoes with jalapeños

4 cups beef stock

1 tbsp. onion powder

1 tbsp. chili powder

1 tsp. cumin garlic powder

1 tsp. Italian seasoning

Salt

A delicious low-carb soup that will kill your hunger dead and keep out the cold.

1. In a large pot, heat the olive oil over a medium heat until hot and cook the sausage. Stir.

2. Chop the green pepper and add to the pot. Stir well. Season with salt and pepper. Add the tomatoes and jalapeños. Stir.

3. Add the spinach on top and cover the pot. When it is wilted, incorporate spices and broth and combine.

4. Cover the pot again and let cook for about 30 minutes (heat medium-low). When it is done, remove the lid and let the soup simmer for around 10 minutes.

NUTRITIONAL INFO PER SERVING

Calories: 525

Fat: 45g

Net Carbs: 4g

Protein: 28g

Mug Cake with Jalapeño

SERVES 1

2 tbsp. almond flour

1 tbsp. flaxseed meal

1 tbsp. butter

1 tbsp. cream cheese

1 egg

1 bacon slice, cooked

½ jalapeño pepper, sliced

½ tsp. baking powder

¼ tsp. salt

Feeling hot, hot, hot? If you like jalapeño peppers, you'll adore this original mug cake.

1. Cook the bacon on a medium heat in a frying pan until crispy.

2. Mix all the ingredients in a container and pour some inside a mug. Microwave for 75 seconds on high.

3. Carefully take out the mug cake out and let cool before eating.

NUTRITIONAL INFO PER SERVING

Calories: 430

Fat: 40g

Net Carbs: 4g

Protein: 17g

Fresh Keto Sandwich

SERVES 1

1 cucumber

1 ½ oz. boursin cheese

Meat of your choice, sliced

Make this fresh sandwich with ingredients easily found in your fridge. Put into your Tupperware, cover, and go!

1. Slice the cucumber in half and scoop out the core and seeds with a spoon. Remove the hard outer skin carefully with a knife.

2. In one side place cheese. In the other side fold meat. Place together to form a sandwich!

NUTRITIONAL INFO PER SERVING

Calories: 195

Fat: 14g

Net Carbs: 8g

Protein: 18g

Original Squash Lasagna

SERVES 12

1 lb. spaghetti squash

3 lb. ground beef

30 slices mozzarella cheese

1 large jar marinara sauce

32 oz. whole milk ricotta cheese

You've probably used spaghetti squash to make spaghetti. But have you tried it for lasagna?

1. Cut the spaghetti squash in two halves, placing them face down onto a baking dish. Add a half inch or so of water. Bake for 45 minutes. When finished, carefully pull out the meat of the squash.

2. In a frying pan, cook the ground beef the meat in a pan and add marinara sauce.

3. In a greased baking pan, place a layer of spaghetti squash, cover with the meat sauce, mozzarella and ricotta. Repeat until the pan is full.

4. Bake for 35 minutes at 375°F.

NUTRITIONAL INFO PER SERVING

Calories: 710

Fat: 60g

Net Carbs: 17g

Protein: 45g

Chili Soup

SERVES 8

2 tbsp. butter, unsalted

2 onions

1 pepper

8 chicken thighs (boneless)

8 slices of bacon

1 tsp. thyme

1 tsp. salt

1 tsp. pepper

1 tbsp. garlic, minced

1 tbsp. coconut flour

3 tbsp. lemon juice

1 cup chicken stock

¼ cup unsweetened coconut milk

3 tbsp. tomato paste

Use your crockpot to make this yummy soup, perfect for a chilly day. Get it? Good.

1. Place the butter in the center of the Crock-Pot.

2. Slice the onion and pepper, and add to the Crock-Pot. Then add the chicken thighs. Top with the bacon slices.

3. Season with salt, pepper, minced garlic, and coconut flour. Add the lemon juice, chicken stocks, coconut milk and tomato paste.

4. Cook on low for 6 hours. When it is done, stir and serve.

NUTRITIONAL INFO PER SERVING

Calories: 395

Fat: 20g

Net Carbs: 8g

Protein: 40g

Chicken Nuggets for Keto Nuts

SERVES 4

1 chicken breast, precooked

½ ounce grated parmesan

2 tbsp. almond flour

½ tsp. baking powder

1 egg

1 tbsp. water

These are quick, and healthier than any nuggets you'll ever buy off the shelf! Try them and see for yourself.

1. Cut the chicken breast into slices and then into bite size pieces. Set aside.

2. Combine the parmesan, almond flour, baking powder, and water. Stir.

3. Cover the chicken pieces into the batter, and then place directly into the hot oil. Remove when golden.

NUTRITIONAL INFO PER SERVING

Calories: 165

Fat: 9g

Net Carbs: 3g

Protein: 25g

Cauliflower Rice with Chicken

SERVES 6

4 chicken breasts

1 packet curry paste

1 cup water

3 tbsp. ghee

½ cup heavy cream

1 head cauliflower

Riced cauliflower is a good option when you have to cook for a lot of people. Also, it is low-carb, and when combined with curry chicken, you'll have a great source of protein.

1. In a large pan, melt the ghee, add the curry, and stir. When combined, add the water, and simmer for 5 minutes.

2. Add the chicken, cover and keep cooking for 20 minutes more. When it is done, add the cream and cook for 5 additional minutes.

3. Separately, prepare the cauliflower rice: chop the head into florets and shred. Sauté in a frying pan with a little butter or olive oil, and then turn to low, covering with a lid. Let it steam for 5-8 minutes.

4. Serve along with the chicken curry.

NUTRITIONAL INFO PER SERVING

Calories: 350

Fat: 16g

Net Carbs: 10g

Protein: 40g

Zucchini Keto Wraps

SERVES 6

1 zucchini

6 oz. soft goat's cheese

1 tbsp. dried mint

1 tsp. dried dill

Salt and pepper

Oil

This one has to be tried to be believed. It serves up to 6 and the mixture of goat's cheese, mint and dill give it a totally unique twist.

1. Cut off the ends of the zucchini. Slice into ⅛-inch slices and brush with oil. Grill on both sides.

2. Mix together the goat's cheese, mint and dill. Divide into 6 pieces.

3. Wrap the cheese pieces with the zucchini slices and secure with a toothpick.

NUTRITIONAL INFO PER SERVING

Calories: 188

Fat: 14g

Net Carbs: 4g

Protein: 15g

Cauliflower Soup with Bacon and Cheddar

SERVES 6

1 head of cauliflower

2 tbsp. olive oil

1 medium onion, diced

4 slices bacon

1 tbsp. minced garlic

1 tsp. thyme

12 oz. aged cheddar

1 oz. parmesan cheese

3 cups chicken broth

¼ cup heavy cream

This soup will warm you up on a cold day. The hearty bacon and cheddar flavor makes it one that even picky eaters will gobble right up!

1. Chop the cauliflower, and place on a foil-lined baking sheet. Sprinkle olive oil and season it with salt and pepper. Bake for 35 minutes at 375°F.

2. In a pot, cook the bacon until crispy. Add diced onion and fry it in the bacon grease. When it is tender, add the garlic and the thyme, and cook for 1 minute or less.

3. Incorporate the chicken broth and cauliflower, and simmer, covered, for 20 minutes.

4. Once time is up, blend the ingredients in a food processor or blender until smooth. Place back into the pot. Add the cheddar and the parmesan cheese, and stir until melted.

5. Finally, add the bacon and the double cream, and mix well. If needed, simmer for 10 minutes more, or until heated.

NUTRITIONAL INFO PER SERVING

Calories: 340

Fat: 26g

Net Carbs: 10g

Protein: 20g

Keto Casserole with Chicken and Bacon

Serves 12

12 chicken thighs

1 small onion

4 celery stalks

24 oz. Jimmy Dean sausage

16 oz. sliced mushrooms

16 oz. frozen cauliflower

7 slices bacon

8 oz. shredded cheddar cheese

16 oz. cream cheese, softened

Paprika

This casserole is a complete meal: chicken, bacon, sausage, veggies and cheese will help you stay full of energy for the rest of your day.

1. In the oven, cook the bacon at 400°F for 15 minutes.

2. Meanwhile, dice the chicken and cook in a frying pan. Remove from pan.

3. Brown the sausage. Once it is done, transfer it to the same bowl as the chicken.

4. Chop the onion and celery, and cook them in the remaining sausage grease until translucent.

5. Defrost the cauliflower, and cut the florets into smaller pieces.

6. In a large bowl, add all the ingredients and mix well. Add the cream cheese and mix well.

7. In large pan, place the mixture and sprinkle the paprika.

8. Bake at 350°F for 30 minutes, covered with a foil. Uncover and cook for an additional 10 minutes.

Nutritional Info per Serving

Calories: 600

Fat: 41g

Net Carbs: 6g

Protein: 53g

Mexican-Style Casserole with Spinach

SERVES 12

1 green pepper

1 onion

20 oz. drained spinach

2 lb. ground pork

2 cans drained diced tomatoes with green chilies

10 tbsp. sour cream

8 oz. mozzarella cheese, shredded

16 oz. cream cheese

4 tsp. taco seasoning

Jalapeños, sliced

This low-carb casserole has all the yummy flavor of tacos, but with a healthier twist.

1. Chop pepper and onion and cook them until translucent. Optional: add diced jalapeños.

2. Place the pepper and onion into a bowl.

3. Cook the spinach by wilting it in a frying pan with a little olive oil. When it is done, add it to the bowl.

4. Cook the ground pork until browned. Season with taco seasoning.

5. Add the diced tomato to the bowl, and incorporate the sour cream, mozzarella and cream cheese. Pour the mixture into a baking dish, and bake at 350°F for 40 minutes.

NUTRITIONAL INFO PER SERVING

Calories: 400

Fat: 30g

Net Carbs: 10g

Protein: 25g

Almond Pizza

SERVES 4

¾ cup almond meal

1½ tsp. baking powder

1½ tsp. granulated sweetener

½ tsp. oregano

¼ tsp. thyme

½ tsp. garlic powder

2 eggs

5 tbsp. butter

½ cup alfredo sauce

4 oz. cheddar cheese

Pizza can be a healthy option when you make the crust with almond meal. Add your favorite toppings and enjoy.

1. Mix the dry ingredients together in a large bowl.
2. Take the eggs (at room temperature) and add to the dry mixture.
3. Melt the butter and incorporate.
4. On a greased pizza pan, spread the crust and pre-cook at 350°F for about 7 minutes.
5. Remove from the oven, and spread the Alfredo Sauce and cheddar cheese on top. Let cook for 5 minutes more.

NUTRITIONAL INFO PER SERVING

Calories: 460

Fat: 45g

Net Carbs: 5g

Protein: 15g

Chicken Salad

SERVES 6

4 chicken breasts

1½ cups cream

4½ oz. celery

4 oz. green peppers

1 ounce green onions

¾ cup sugar free sweet relish

¾ cup mayo

3 eggs, hard-boiled

Fresh and nutritious, this easy recipe can be part of a whole meal or served as a side.

1. Place the chicken in an oven-safe pan, and cover it with cream. Cook for 40-60 minutes at 350°F. When it is done, let cool. Discard the liquid.

2. Chop the celery, pepper and onions, and combine them in a bowl. Dice the chicken and add too.

3. Add chopped hardboiled eggs and mix gently.

3. Divide into 6 containers.

NUTRITIONAL INFO PER SERVING

Calories: 415

Fat: 24g

Net Carbs: 4g

Protein: 40g

Keto Chicken Thighs

SERVES 6

16 chicken thighs (boneless skinless)

2 cups water

8 oz. cheddar cheese, shredded

24 oz. spinach

Salt and pepper

Garlic powder

Three main ingredients. Thirty minutes. One delicious dinner. You can also divide into containers for a yummy lunch option!

1. Bake the chicken thighs in a covered pan with 2 cups of water at 350°F for 20 minutes. Remove and let cool.

2. Break the chicken into pieces, adding the spinach, cheese, and seasonings.

NUTRITIONAL INFO PER SERVING

Calories: 390

Fat: 25g

Net Carbs: 4g

Protein: 47g

BBQ Chicken Soup

SERVES 4

3 medium chicken thighs

2 tsp. chili seasoning

2 tbsp. olive oil

1½ cups chicken broth

1½ cups beef broth

BBQ sauce

¼ cup reduced sugar ketchup

¼ cup tomato paste

2 tbsp. Dijon mustard

1 tbsp. soy sauce

1 tbsp. hot sauce

2½ tsp. liquid smoke

1 tsp. Worcestershire sauce

1½ tsp. garlic powder

1 tsp. onion powder

1 tsp. chili powder

1 tsp. red chili flakes

1 tsp. cumin

¼ cup butter

Salt and pepper

A low-carb soup that comes with an original BBQ flavor. A surefire winner every lunchtime.

1. Take the chicken thighs and de-bone. Reserve the bones. Season with favorite chili seasoning. Bake for 50 minutes at 400°F on a baking tray with foil.

2. In a pot, place olive oil and set on medium high heat. Once it is hot, add the chicken bones. Cook them for 5 minutes and add the broth. Season with salt and pepper.

3. When chicken is done, take off the skin. Incorporate the fat from the chicken into the broth and stir.

4. Make the BBQ Sauce: combine all the already mentioned ingredients for the sauce. Add it to the pot and stir. Let it simmer 20-30 minutes.

5. Emulsify all the fats and liquid together with an immersion blender. Shred the chicken and incorporate into the soup. Cook for 10-20 minutes more.

NUTRITIONAL INFO PER SERVING

Calories: 490

Fat: 38g

Net Carbs: 4.5g

Protein: 25g

Keto Pork Stew

SERVES 4

1 lb. pork shoulder, cooked and sliced

2 tsp. chili powder

2 tsp. cumin

1 tsp. garlic, minced

½ tsp. salt

½ tsp. pepper

1 tsp. paprika

1 tsp. oregano

¼ tsp. cinnamon

2 bay leaves

6 oz. button mushrooms

½ jalapeño, sliced

½ onion, medium

½ sliced green bell pepper

½ sliced red bell pepper

Juice of ½ a lime

2 cups gelatinous bone broth

2 cups chicken broth

½ cup strong coffee

¼ cup tomato paste

This stew is perfect for when the rain is drizzling down the window outside, and you the family fancies a little pick-me-up.

1. Dice the vegetables, and sauté them in a pan lined with olive oil over high heat. Remove from heat when browned.

2. Chop pork and put into a slow cooker with mushrooms, bone broth, chicken broth and coffee.

3. Incorporate spices and vegetables as well and mix. Place the lid. Cook for 4-10 hours on low.

NUTRITIONAL INFO PER SERVING

Calories: 385

Fat: 29g

Net Carbs: 6.4g

Protein: 20g

Keto Enchilada Soup

SERVES 4

- 3 tbsp. olive oil
- 3 diced celery stalks
- 1 medium diced red bell pepper
- 2 tsp. minced garlic
- 1 cup diced tomatoes
- 2 tsp. cumin
- 1 tsp. oregano
- 1 tsp. chili powder
- ½ tsp. cayenne pepper
- ½ cup chopped cilantro
- 4 cups chicken broth
- 8 oz. cream cheese
- 6 oz. shredded chicken
- Juice of ½ a lime

This soup is both spicy and creamy, and so delicious that you'll forget all about how healthy it is.

1. In a hot pan with olive oil, sauté the celery and pepper. When the celery starts to become tender, add the tomatoes and cook for 2-3 minutes longer.

2. Incorporate the spices. Add the chicken broth and cilantro, letting it boil. Reduce to a low heat, and simmer for about 20 minutes.

3. Add the cheese and boil again. Reduce to a low heat and simmer for 25 minutes more.

4. Add the shredded chicken with the lime juice. Stir.

5. Season with cilantro and serve.

NUTRITIONAL INFO PER SERVING

Calories: 345

Fat: 31g

Net Carbs: 6.3g

Protein: 13g

Grilled Cheese Sandwich

SERVES 1

2 eggs

2 tbsp. almond flour

1 ½ tbsp. psyllium husk powder

½ tsp. baking powder

2 tbsp. soft butter

2 oz. cheddar cheese

1 tbsp. butter

A crispy option for lunch, and even better with soup on the side, this little number will have you drooling.

1. Mix the eggs, almond flour, psyllium husk powder, baking powder and butter to make the bun. It should be very thick. Place the mixture into a square container and let it sit to level itself. Microwave for 90 seconds.

2. When it is cooked, remove and slice in half. Place the cheese between the bun, and fry in a pan with melted butter over a medium heat.

NUTRITIONAL INFO PER SERVING

Calories: 794

Fat: 72g

Net Carbs: 5g

Protein: 30g

Keto Caprese Salad

SERVES 1

1 tomato

6 oz. fresh mozzarella cheese

¼ cup chopped fresh basil

3 tbsp. olive oil

Freshly cracked black pepper

Salt

This simple recipe takes a quick 5 minutes, but is chock-full of fresh flavor.

1. Put the fresh basil in a food processor with some oil. Blend until it forms a paste.

2. Slice the tomatoes and chop the mozzarella. On the top of each tomato, lay the mozzarella and basil paste. Season with olive oil, black pepper and salt.

NUTRITIONAL INFO PER SERVING

Calories: 407

Fat: 38g

Net Carbs: 3.7g

Protein: 16g

Asian Salad

SERVES 1

1 packet shirataki noodles

2 tbsp. coconut oil

1 cucumber

1 spring onion

¼ tbsp. red pepper flakes

1 tbsp. sesame oil

1 tbsp. rice vinegar

1 tsp. sesame seeds

Salt and pepper

Cucumbers are the fresh tasting stars of this dish. Includes the crunch of fried shirataki noodles, and a slightly spicy flavoring to make it more interesting.

1. Wash the shirataki noodles. Strain off all the excess water. Let them dry on a paper towel.

2. In a pan, heat the coconut oil over a medium-high, and fry the noodles for 5-7 minutes. Remove and set on a paper towel to cool.

3. Peel and slice the cucumber. Arrange on a plate, and add the rest of the ingredients, sprinkling over the cucumber. Let chill for 30 minutes in the fridge.

4. Top with fried shirataki noodles.

NUTRITIONAL INFO PER SERVING

Calories: 418

Fat: 45g

Net Carbs: 8g

Protein: 3g

Vegetarian Curry

SERVES 2

4 tbsp. coconut oil

¼ onion, chopped

1 tsp. garlic, minced

1 cup broccoli florets

Spinach

1 tbsp. red curry paste

½ cup coconut cream (or coconut milk)

2 tsp. soy sauce

1 tsp. ginger

2 tsp. fish sauce

This red curry combines unique flavors and leaves you with an easy recipe that your taste buds will love!

1. On a medium-high heat, add the coconut oil to a pan. Once it is hot, sauté the onions until browned. Add the garlic. Turn to a medium-low heat and add the broccoli. Stir.

2. Once the broccoli is partially cooked, add the curry paste. Let it cook for 1 minute.

3. Add the spinach. When it is cooked, add coconut cream and coconut oil.

3. Mix and add the soy sauce, ginger and fish sauce. Simmer for approximately 10 minutes.

NUTRITIONAL INFO PER SERVING

Calories: 395

Fat: 40g

Net Carbs: 7g

Protein: 6g

FREE BONUS GUIDE:
Top 10 Keto Diet Mistakes

We hope you enjoy making your way through the delicious meals contained in this cookbook, and want to offer you a little something extra to ensure you stay safe and maximize your results.

With our free bonus guide you will learn the top 10 mistakes people make when cooking keto, and discover exactly how to avoid them for yourself. Curious? Use the link below to see it now!

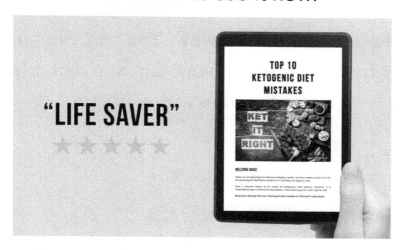

Visit **http://geni.us/ketomistakes** to get your copy now!

Like This Book?

This is Buster, and he'd really love to know what you thought!

If you got value from this book, or the free bonus guide, it would be amazing if you could visit your Amazon order history to leave a quick review. You can even upload a picture of your favorite recipe! Oh, and don't forget to share the love with a friend!

CPSIA information can be obtained
at www.ICGtesting.com
Printed in the USA
BVHW01s1942180618
519355BV00007B/60/P

9 781544 720333